ROLF
MILONAS

FANTASEX

A Perigee Book

Perigee Books
are published by
The Putnam Publishing Group
200 Madison Avenue
New York, New York 10016

Published simultaneously in Canada by
General Publishing Co. Limited, Toronto.

Library of Congress Cataloging in
Publication Data

Milonas, Rolf.
Fantasex.
1. Sex customs.   2. Sex role.   3. Sexual
fantasies.
I. Title.
HQ21.M65   1983   306.7   83-8258
ISBN 0-399-50839-2

Book design by Jan White

First Perigee Printing, 1983
Printed in the United States of America
5 6 7 8 9

To Eros and Aphrodite

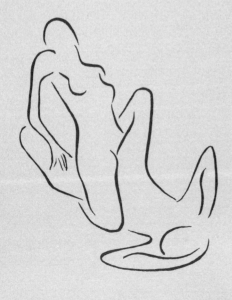

INTRODUCTION

The Fantasex games are designed for adult couples who are fond of each other, have access to privacy and would enjoy some experimentation and adventure in their love-making.

The games offer the Players the choice of practically infinite combinations of plays through which they can communicate and offer pleasure to themselves and their partners.

By projecting themselves into the imaginary situations and roles, and by allowing the rules of the game, or pure chance, to make some of the basic decisions for them, the Players can experience interesting and unusual relationships and perhaps find the freedom to do some of the things they have always wanted to do together but somehow have never actually experienced.

The games are non-competitive and non-adversary and there is no winner or loser. The goal is simply the uninhibited enjoyment derived from sharing—the giving and receiving of pleasure.

The material in the book was selected to cover a range of common indulgences and fantasies, and it will be up to the Players to censor that which may prevent them from appreciating the game as fun. Should it become unpleasant or prove a turn-off to either, stop the game.

GETTING
READY
TO PLAY

Ideally, plan ahead together
and relish the anticipation of playing the game.

Soak in a hot bath, treat yourselves
to a special dab of perfume or after-shave
lotion, enjoy a leisurely but light meal.

Set the mood with soft background music,
candlelight, and light some incense.

Take the phone off the hook, nestle into
a cozy couch or among some pillows on the floor.

Take your time and relax
with a glass of wine and perhaps a smoke.

THE GAME PLANS

The Players must agree
on one of the four Game Plans which they
will follow during the playing of the Game.
These Plans simply determine how some
of the critical decisions are reached.

Plan I—*Cooperative Plan*
All decisions are made by mutual consent.

Plan II—*Male Dominant Plan*
He makes all the decisions.

Plan III—*Female Dominant Plan*
She makes all the decisions.

Plan IV—*Pure Chance Plan*
The numbers they choose will make the decisions
for the Players.

DRESS UP OPTIONS

The fun of make-believe can be enhanced by dressing up or dressing down for the game using props that can be found in anybody's closet. One may start fully or partially dressed, one may be fully dressed but omit part or all of the undergarments, or perhaps find something that is tight, revealing or transparent.

There is a whole range of tactile sensations that can be explored through the use of materials such as fur, feathers, silk, leather, rubber and velvet. Special costumes can be easily fashioned from scarves, belts, towels, sheets and body stockings, while accessories such as garter belts, athletic supporters, boots and wigs can help any improvisation.

Interesting variations can be made by wearing the clothing of the other, and both Players should most certainly take advantage of the effects of perfumes, after-shave lotions, powder and make-up, not to mention the imaginative use of jewelry.

FANTASEX GAME VARIATIONS

GROUP FANTASEX
Three or more Players can play by following the basic
directions, with minor variations. They must modify the
fantasy situations in such a way as to include the additional
Players, or they must select an additional character from the
Roles list. In either case, the extra participants must be
logically incorporated into the game.

SEMI-SOLITAIRE FANTASEX
Either Player makes his or her selections, in secret, without
telling the other, and lives the fantasy when they make love.

SOLITAIRE FANTASEX
A Player can make any selections he wishes and can happily
play the game by simply fantasizing alone.

INSTRUCTIONS FOR PLAYING ROLE FANTASEX

THE SECTIONS OF THE BOOK

The book is divided into several sections which can be easily recognized by leafing through. For the game of Role Fantasex, the Players use the sections entitled "Roles," "Plays" and "Positions."

THE ROLES

A list of male and female character roles is given in the "Roles" section which follows the introductory material. After reviewing the many options and considering different role juxtapositions, the Players find any combination of characters that appeals to their mood and whimsy.

The Roles may be modified by attributing social, racial or temperamental characteristics to them.

If they are playing the Cooperative Game Plan, they can make the selection together. If they have decided on the Male or Female Dominant Game Plan, one Player will determine both their Roles. Or if the Players have chosen the Pure Chance Game Plan, each Player picks a number from 1 to 32; they must then find the corresponding number on the His and Hers "Roles" pages.

ROLES

The Players will assume these selected or assigned Roles, and relate to each other with this new personality during the rest of the game.

THE PLAYS

With the Roles established, the Players proceed to the "Plays" section of the book. From the options, the Players following the Cooperative Game Plan each select at least *one* Play situation. If they have selected a Male or Female Dominant Game Plan, one Player will choose at least *two* Plays. Or if the Players have chosen the Pure Chance Game Plan, each player picks a number from 1 to 30; they must then find the corresponding number in the "Plays" section of the book, and proceed with those Plays.

The Players must follow all the Play instructions before concluding the game.

THE·POSITIONS

Next, if they are playing the Cooperative Game Plan, either Player may choose any one Position from the "Positions" section of the book.

If they are playing the Male or Female Dominant Game Plan, one Player picks the Position.

If the Players have chosen the Pure Chance Game Plan, either Player may pick a number from 1 to 22. They must then find the corresponding number in the "Positions" section of the book, and proceed with that Position.

No matter which Game Plan has been played, the position chosen is the one that must be followed to consummate the game.

THE PROCEDURE

If they wish, the Players may dress up or dress down as befits their assumed roles. In any case, with all the decisions made, the Players relax and perhaps have another glass of wine while they fantasize together and create the appropriate setting into which they will project their new personalities and relationship. They let their imaginary characters start to take over and gradually lead them into the exciting world of make-believe as they begin playing the game.

ROLES

FOR
USE
WHEN
PLAYING
THE
ROLE
FANTASEX
GAME

ROLES

EACH
PLAYER
GETS
ONE
ROLE

FOR
USE
WHEN
PLAYING
THE
ROLE
FANTASEX
GAME

ROLES

EACH
PLAYER
GETS
ONE
ROLE

HIS ROLES

13 BLIND GENIUS

15 PLAYBOY

32 TV ÀNCHORMAN

14 HAIRDRESSER

8 SLAVE BOY

25 HEADMASTER

6 PRIEST

4 SECRET AGENT

12 DELIVERY BOY

19 MASKED STRANGER

18 FAMOUS ATHLETE

7 ARAB SHEIK

11 HUNTED GUERILLA LEADER

17 GIGOLO

3 GYNECOLOGIST

16 NAZI OFFICER

1 HIRED KILLER

31 CHARISMATIC POLITICIAN

30 PSYCHIATRIST

20 GODFATHER

21 ROCK STAR

5 TRUCK DRIVER

22 FAMOUS MOVIE STAR

29 TRAVELING SALESMAN

23 PIRATE

27 PENNILESS ARTIST

10 MALE PROSTITUTE

9 BEST FRIEND'S HUSBAND

2 COWBOY

24 HOSTAGE

26 PORNO MOVIE DIRECTOR

28 BEACHCOMBER

ROLES

HER
ROLES

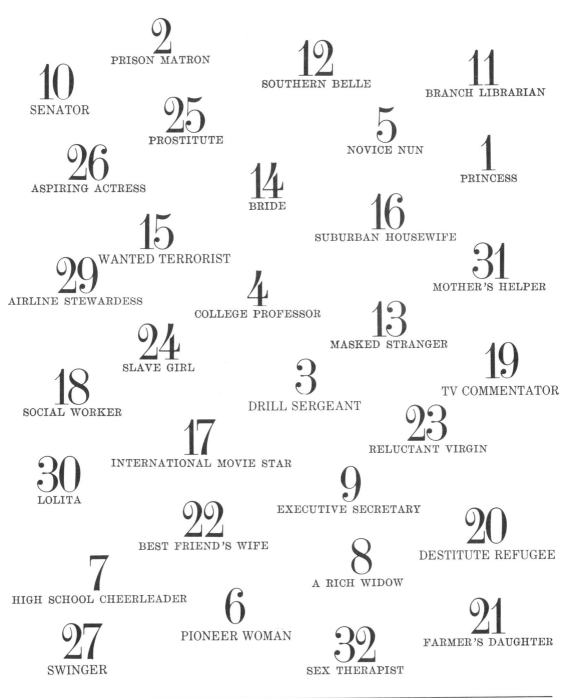

2 PRISON MATRON

12 SOUTHERN BELLE

11 BRANCH LIBRARIAN

10 SENATOR

25 PROSTITUTE

5 NOVICE NUN

1 PRINCESS

26 ASPIRING ACTRESS

14 BRIDE

16 SUBURBAN HOUSEWIFE

15 WANTED TERRORIST

31 MOTHER'S HELPER

29 AIRLINE STEWARDESS

4 COLLEGE PROFESSOR

13 MASKED STRANGER

24 SLAVE GIRL

19 TV COMMENTATOR

18 SOCIAL WORKER

3 DRILL SERGEANT

23 RELUCTANT VIRGIN

30 LOLITA

17 INTERNATIONAL MOVIE STAR

9 EXECUTIVE SECRETARY

22 BEST FRIEND'S WIFE

20 DESTITUTE REFUGEE

7 HIGH SCHOOL CHEERLEADER

8 A RICH WIDOW

27 SWINGER

6 PIONEER WOMAN

32 SEX THERAPIST

21 FARMER'S DAUGHTER

PLAYERS
MUST
SELECT
AND
PLAY
AT
LEAST
ONE
PLAY

PLAYS

FOR
USE
WHEN
PLAYING
EITHER
ROLE
OR
SITUATION
FANTASEX

PLAYERS
MUST
SELECT
AND
PLAY
AT
LEAST
ONE

PLAY

PLAYS

FOR
USE
WHEN
PLAYING
EITHER
ROLE
OR
SITUATION
FANTASEX

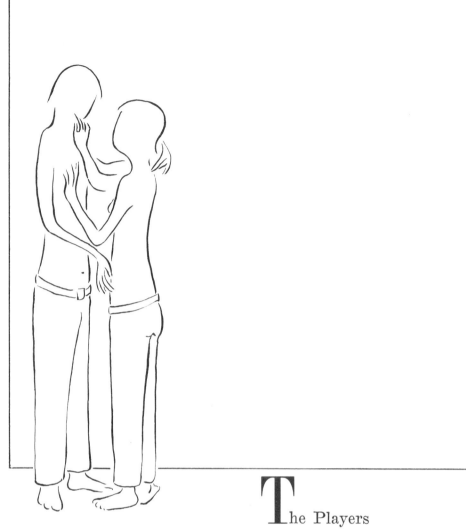

The Players
dance closely, touching only
with the tips of their fingers, which are used
to ever so gently caress
while helping the other to undress.
Lips and tongues explore
each new surface as it becomes exposed,
bodies still only brushing lightly
so that each Player can savor
the sensitivity and the texture of the other's skin,
until finally, they terminate the Play
with a close embrace.

1

PLAY

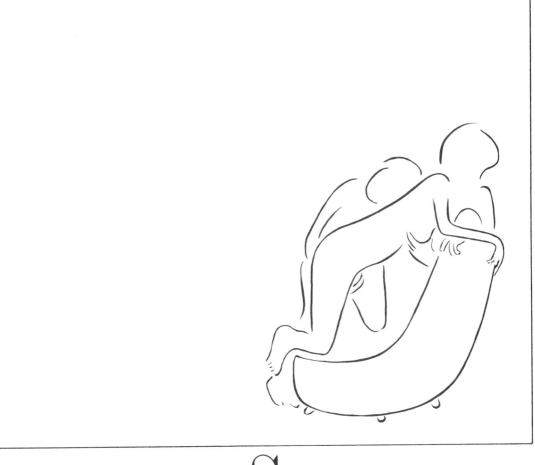

She kneels
on a chair with arms resting on the back
her legs slightly apart;
from behind, with one hand fondling her breasts,
he explores her genitals with the other.
He may shift from the breasts if
both hands are needed below
to enhance her pleasure
and he may take advantage of her position
by entering her experimentally,
providing he is sure to withdraw
before losing control.

2
PLAY

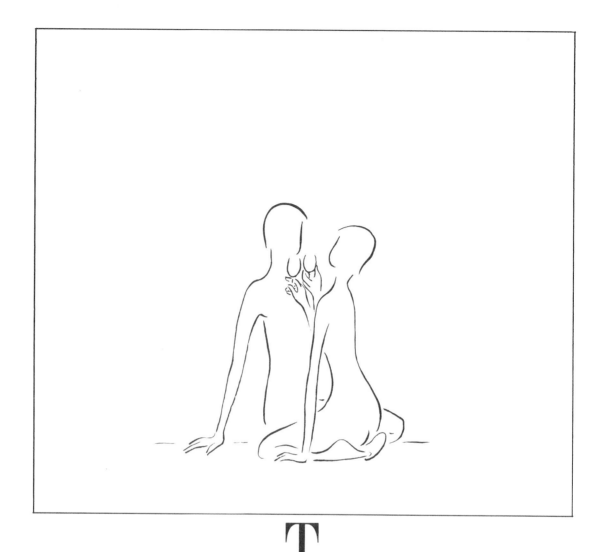

The Players
take their drinks and candle
to the bathroom,
where they spread a blanket on the floor
and get the room steamy by turning on the shower.
They wait
until they glisten with perspiration
before caressing and enjoying each other's stickiness.
They conclude this Play in a sixty-nine position,
followed by an eventful shower,
before they return to continue the game in
some other place where it is dry.

3

PLAY

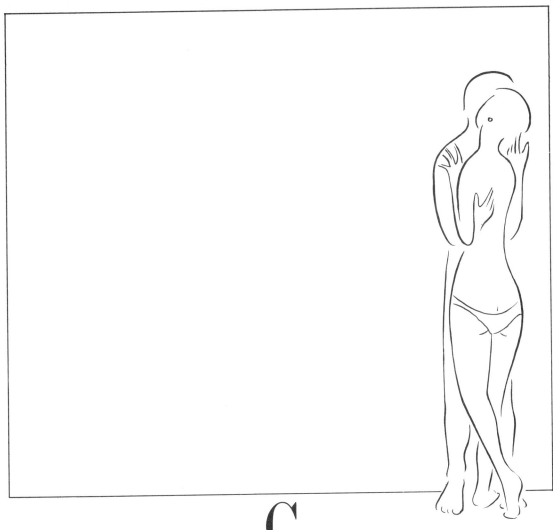

Comfortably close,
the Players take turns
caressing
the many sensitive parts
above the other's shoulders.
Starting with the neck and throat,
they move behind the ear, the lobes, the ears themselves,
the chin, the lips, the nose, the eyes,
and then the mouth, both outside and in,
using fingers, lips, tongue and teeth
as delicate tools
to stimulate excitement and pleasure.

4

PLAY

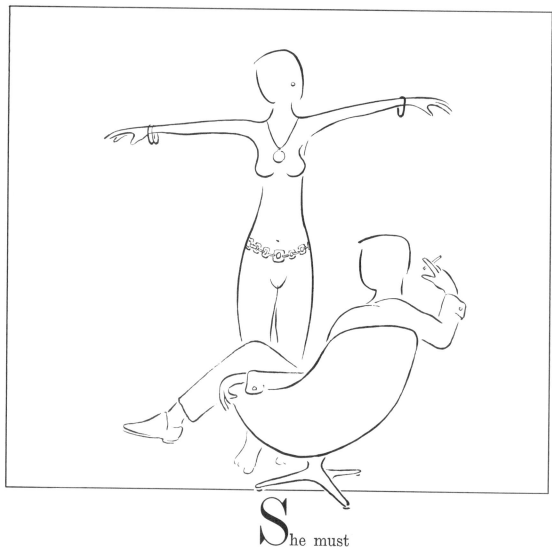

She must
stand and obediently move as he may direct so that
he may enjoy looking at and touching her every part.
He may dress or undress her,
decorate her with lipstick, order her to dance
or do anything that will intrigue and amuse him.
She may not move or touch him
unless he gives her instructions,
but he may handle her body in any way
exclusively for selfish pleasure
as long as it doesn't cause
his premature ejaculation.

5

PLAY

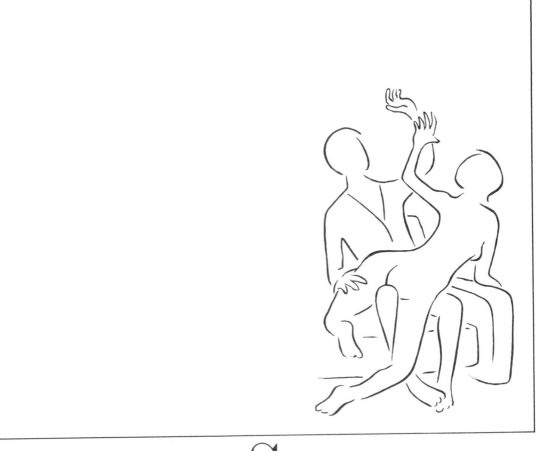

She incorporates
into their fantasy her confession of
a shocking imaginary sin
which she claims to have committed,
drawing perhaps on something she read
in some outrageous porno material.
She begs his forgiveness
and depending on their roles or situations
she requests or he demands her punishment.
He lays her across his lap
and gives her
a sound spanking.

6

PLAY

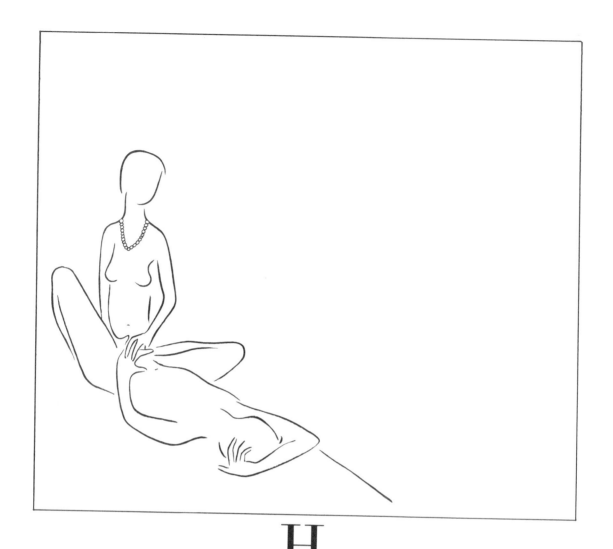

H
e relaxes
on a blanket spread on the kitchen table, and
she treats him to a sensuous massage with cold cream.
Moving from his back to his front,
she gradually arrives
at his genitals.
Lovingly she caresses and explores them in great detail
as he guides her fingers with his to specific areas,
telling her exactly
how and what
he would like her to do
to create the most pleasurable sensations.

7
PLAY

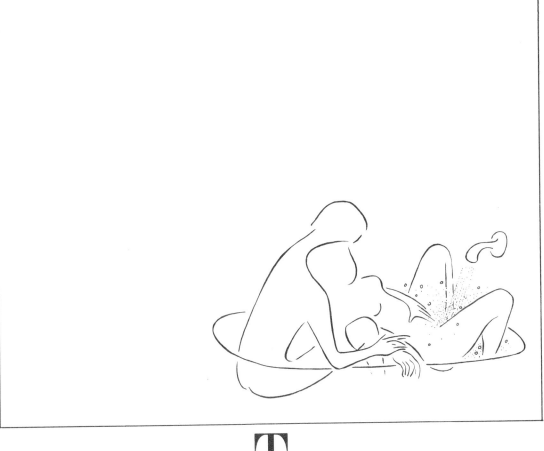

The Players

take a shower together and enjoy
handling each other's wet and slippery bodies.
After a while,
with the tub unplugged, they turn on
comfortably warm water from the faucet.
She sits with her legs apart, facing the stream
and allows the water to stimulate her exposed clitoris.
While he supports her from the back,
he sensuously lathers her breasts with soap
and continues playing until the water
brings her to an orgasm.

8

PLAY

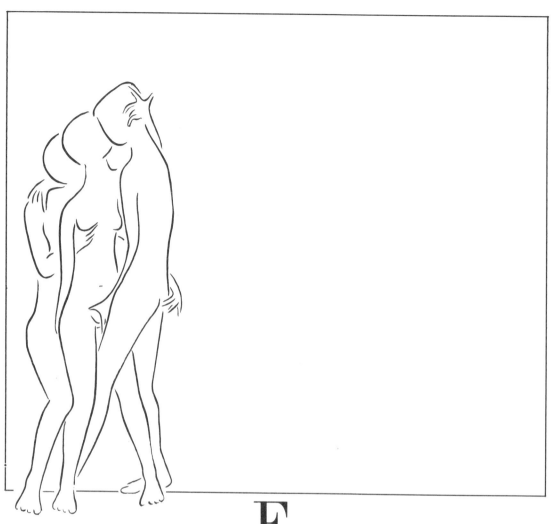

Expanding on
their imaginary relationship,
the Players invent a Second Man
who will have to participate in the fantasy they share.
After discussing
just how they will include and use him
in their fantasy
they close their eyes and caress each other
while either or both
pretend
that the other's hands and mouth
really belong to the imagined Second Man.

9

PLAY

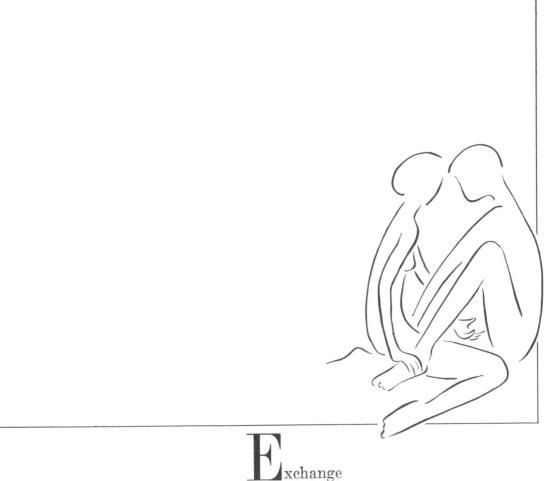

Exchange
this Play for another
unless it is very warm. Use
a towel to protect the furniture.
Each Player passes an ice cube
over the other's body,
enjoying the reactions.
When ready to consummate the game,
and at the critical moment
each presses an ice cube to the other's genitals
to enhance the intensity
of the orgasm.

10

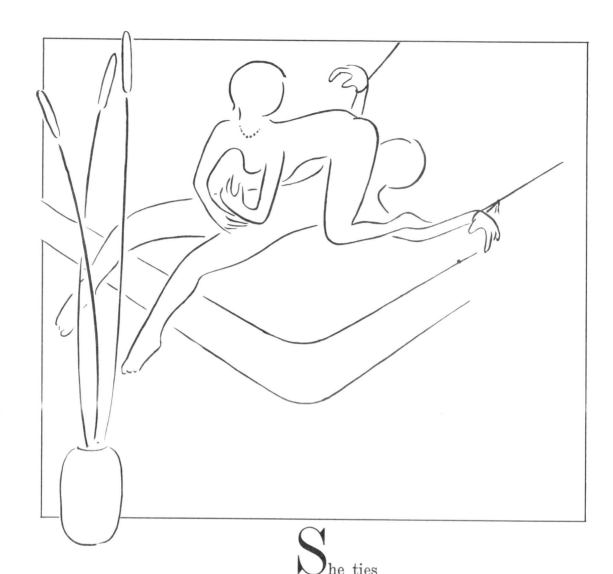

She ties
his wrists and ankles with ribbons
and secures him spread-eagle to the bed, leaving him
vulnerably exposed.
Straddling him, she lazily toys with his penis
to her heart's content,
selfishly taking care that he is not prematurely wasted.
Since there is no reason she should have to wait,
she may move over to his head
and inspire him to use his mouth and tongue creatively,
enjoying him until she is ready
before freeing him of his bonds.

11

PLAY

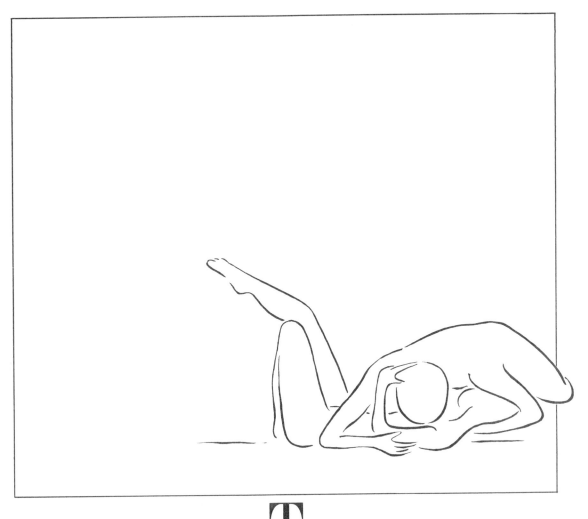

The Players
find something tasty in the pantry or refrigerator,
something they know that
the other will like,
such as beluga caviar, whipped cream or grape jelly
(but certainly not all three).
They spread the delicacy on each other's
breasts and navels and other interesting parts,
and when they are ready
they relish each other
making certain that absolutely
nothing is wasted.

12

PLAY

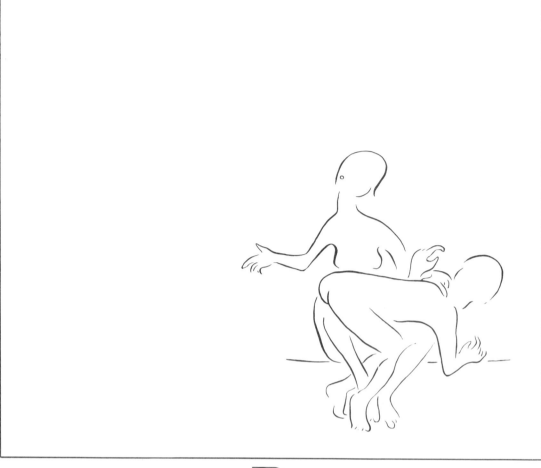

Based on
something he has read, say in Marquis de Sade,
he invents a wild story
which he incorporates into their fantasy,
confessing
in great detail just how he actively participated
in a strange erotic adventure.
He begs her forgiveness and
depending on their roles or situations
he requests or she demands his punishment.
She lays him across her lap
and gives him a sound spanking.

13

PLAY

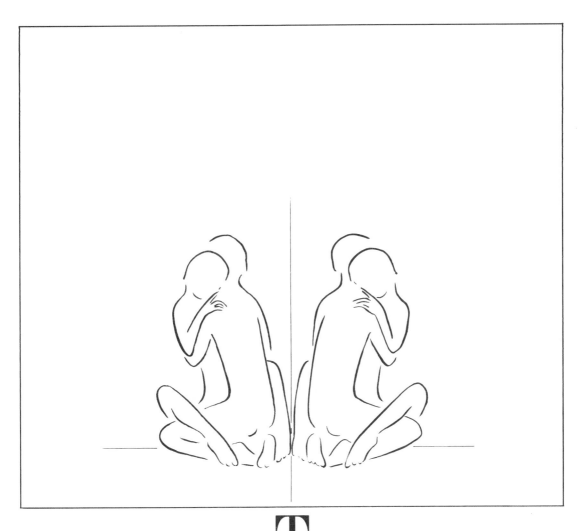

Together

the Players select six Positions
from the back of the book.
They spread a blanket and some cushions in front
of a full-length mirror.
They play while watching themselves,
and as they assume different positions,
he enters her briefly in each
using great self-control.
When they are finally ready
to consummate the game,
they return to the mirror and watch themselves perform.

14
PLAY

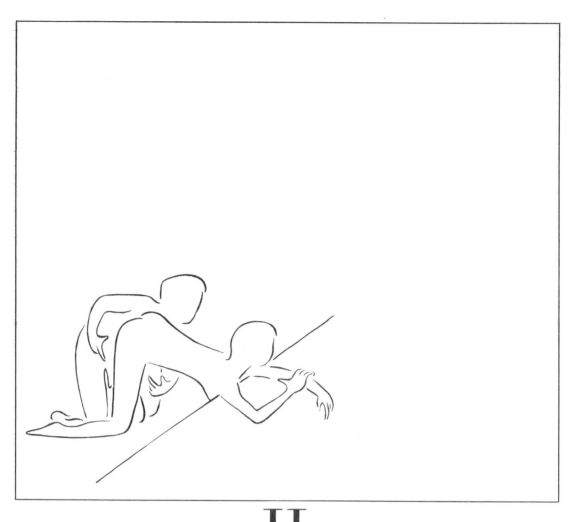

H e leans
her over a table or a bed and lubricates her anus
with baby oil or petroleum jelly, before
he gently inserts his finger.
When she is completely relaxed, he withdraws,
only to re-enter her from behind once more,
this time with his penis.
Moving slowly and gently and without a sudden thrust,
he responds to her every move,
as he fondles her breasts and toys with her clitoris.
Before resuming vaginal contact
he excuses himself and washes.

15

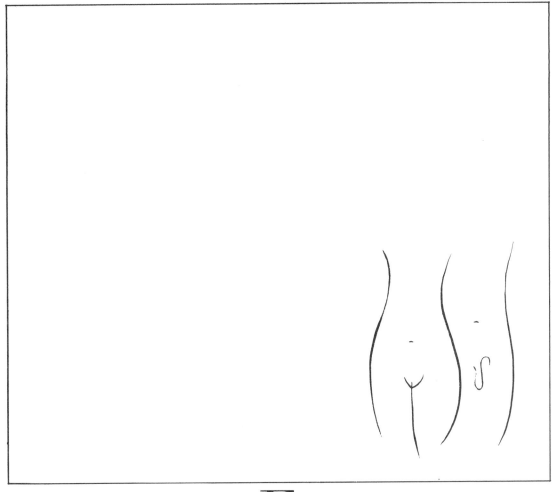

Either Player
may reject this Play and exchange it for another,
or either may proceed
independently
by going to the bath
to shave off the pubic hair.
It will grow back in a few weeks
though it may itch slightly for a while.
After applying powder
the Players enhance
their newly found nakedness by covering themselves
before returning to the game.

16

PLAY

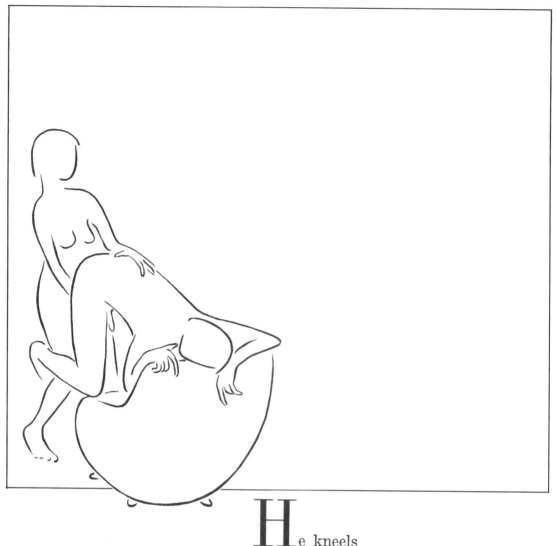

H e kneels
on a chair, arms on the back, legs slightly apart.
From behind, she caresses his buttocks and legs
and centers her attention on
his vulnerable parts.
She plays with him creatively using both hands
and after a while, if her nails are not too long,
she lubricates one finger with petroleum jelly and
carefully enters his anus, gently exploring
while holding on to his scrotum
to firmly control
his squirmings.

17

PLAY

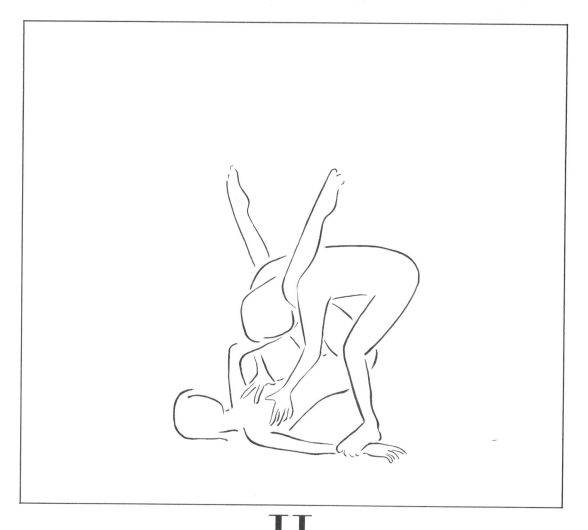

He strips
her naked before he undresses and applies baby oil
to her body to make her slippery all over.
Against her will,
he then attacks and tries to take her
in any way he can
as she struggles hard to avoid penetration.
When he succeeds, he must immediately withdraw,
so that they can repeat the Play
as many times as they like it,
he forcing her each time
into a different position.

18
PLAY

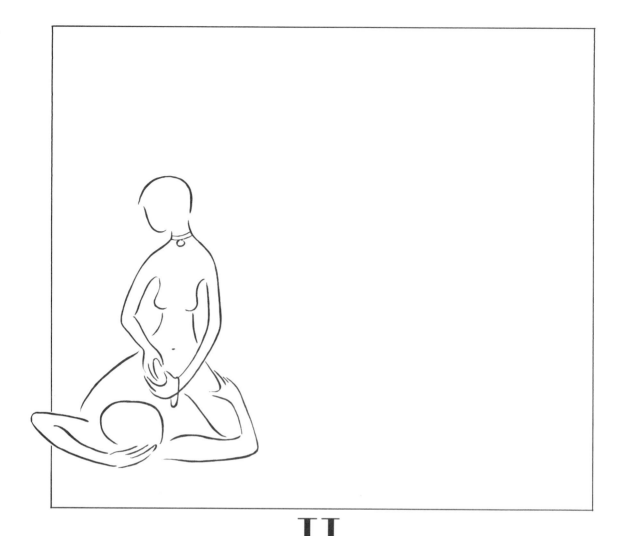

He lies
on the carpet among some pillows,
and after covering him with fleeting kisses,
she caresses his erection.
At her pleasure
she lowers herself on him
as often and in as many positions as she likes,
never staying long enough
to lose him prematurely.
She may lean over and allow him
to enjoy her breasts
and may encourage him to actively participate.

19
PLAY

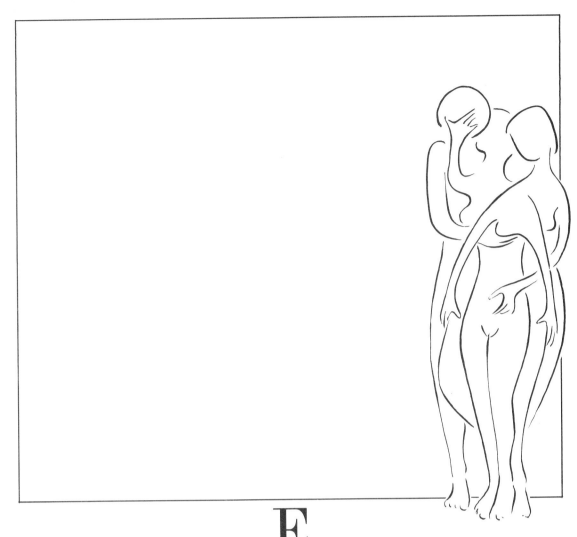

Expanding on
their imaginary relationship,
the Players invent a Second Woman
who will have to participate in the fantasy they share.
After discussing
just how they will include and use her
in their fantasy,
they close their eyes and caress each other
while either or both
pretend
that the other's hands and mouth
really belong to the imagined Second Woman.

20

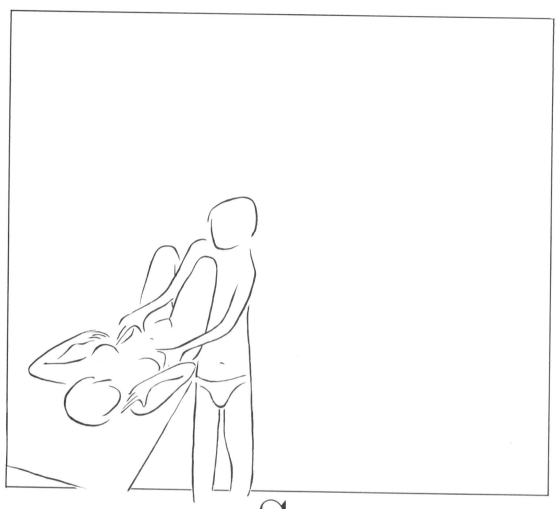

She relaxes
on a blanket spread on the kitchen or dining room table
and he treats her to a sensuous massage with cold cream.
Moving from her back to her front
he gradually arrives
at her genitals.
Lovingly he caresses and explores them in great detail
as she guides his fingers with hers to specific areas
telling him exactly
how and what
she would like him to do
to create the most pleasurable sensations.

21

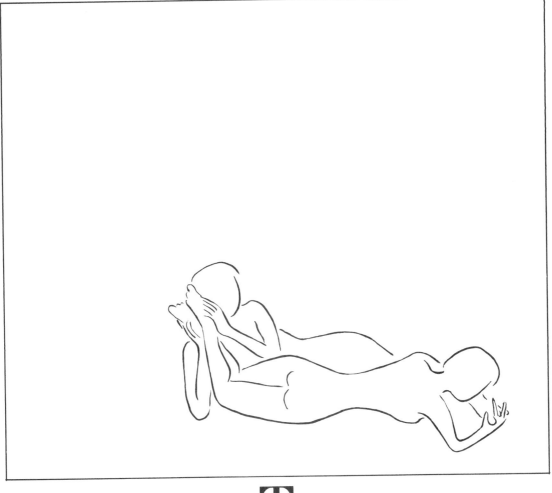

The Players
lie close to each other,
their heads at opposite sides,
and restrict their attention
to each other's feet.
They make love to instep, sole, heel, ankle
and one by one, to every toe.
With fingers, lips, teeth, tongue and genitals
they use contacts from light brushings to firm squeezes
to stimulate,
enjoy
and give pleasure to the other.

22

PLAY

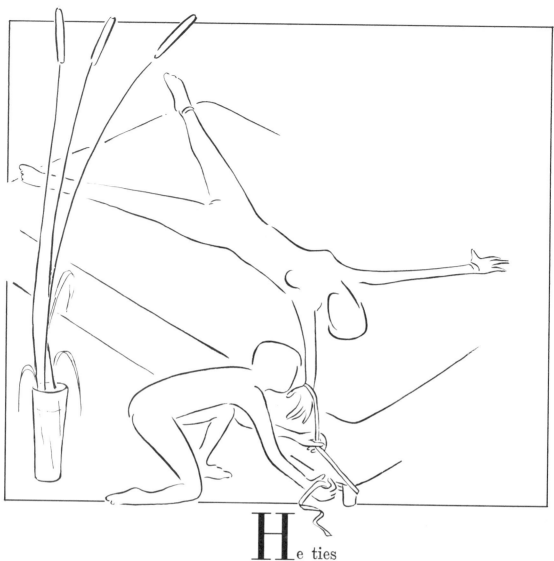

He ties
her wrists and ankles with ribbons
and secures her spread-eagle to the bed, leaving her
vulnerably exposed.
He then tortures her mercilessly with kisses,
tickles nipples and clitoris, perhaps using a feather,
and does everything that he knows that will excite her.
He may briefly enter her
just for fun,
but he must withdraw in time for them to continue playing.
For safety's sake
he unties her immediately after the play.

23
PLAY

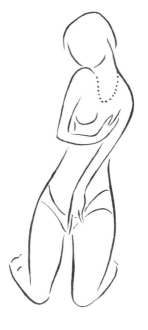

He must
give his word of honor
to remain seated and not attack her.
As he watches,
she slowly strips off her clothing,
moving and caressing herself seductively,
perhaps dancing to background music.
She concentrates entirely on the pleasure of her own body
as she masturbates
either ostentatiously
or in disregard of her lover
who is forced to watch.

24

PLAY

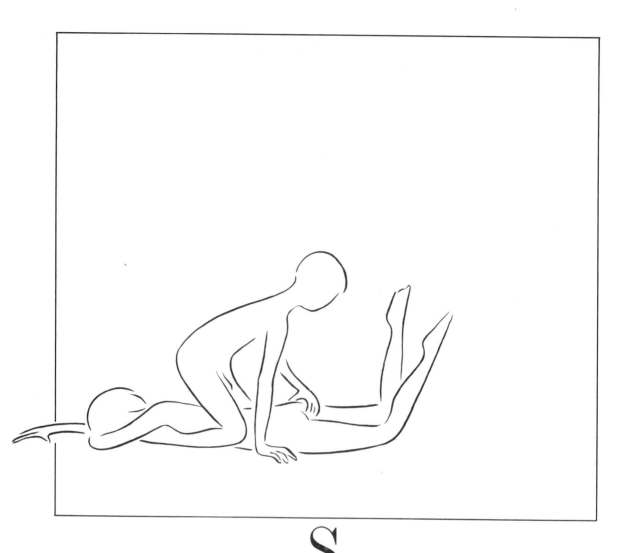

She lies
face down and he kneels by her side.
He strokes her back, lightly scratching and massaging
until he gets to her buttocks
which he roughly manipulates,
occasionally reaching teasingly between her legs.
If she squirms or makes ungrateful noises,
he will punish her
by spanking her,
increasing the blows until she manages to wiggle away.
She then requires him to assume the same position
so that she may revenge herself in kind.

25

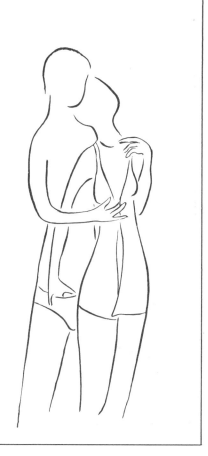

The Players

put on clothing that won't be harmed when wet.
Taking along the candle, they move to the bath
where fully dressed
they step into the shower.
They soap each other through the clinging clothes
and play, enjoying
the wet look and sensations.
Finally, after stripping each other
and drying off,
the Players return to the game
provocatively wrapped in towels.

26

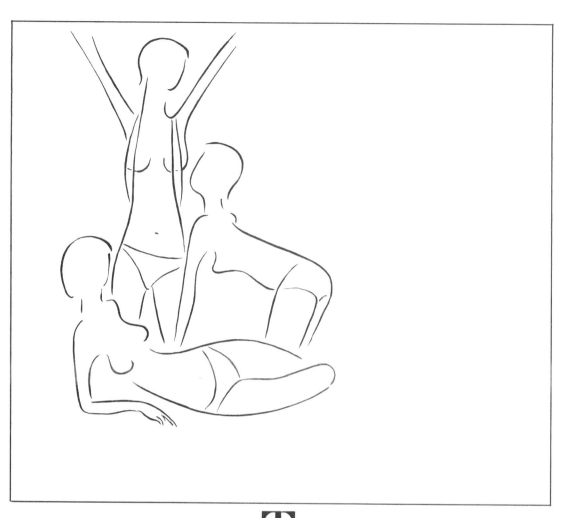

To show off
the many beautiful and exciting shapes
that a woman's breasts can assume
she moves her body for him
by leaning forward, bending backward
and twisting her torso.
Concentrating on her breasts and armpits
he enjoys and gives pleasure by using
fingers, hands, face, hair, lips, tongue and penis
in an attempt to bring her to orgasm
without
touching any other part of her body.

27

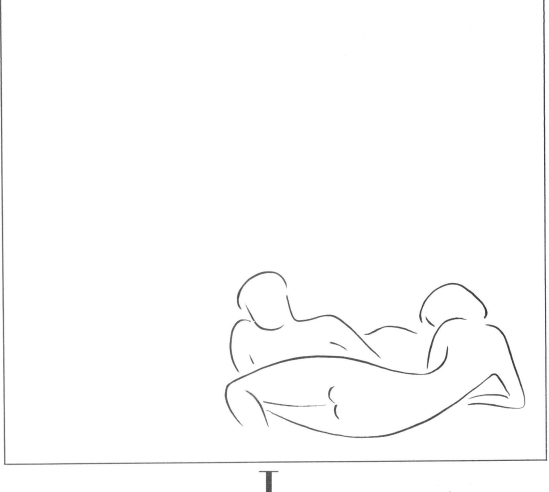

Lying intimately
side by side, with heads on opposite ends,
the Players concentrate their caresses
to restricted body parts.
He plays with her most intimate areas
without touching her clitoris
while she restricts her toying to his scrotum.
No matter how tempting it becomes for both
neither may otherwise touch the other
until finally,
as reward for having endured this torturous pleasure,
the lovers are left to their own devices.

28

PLAY

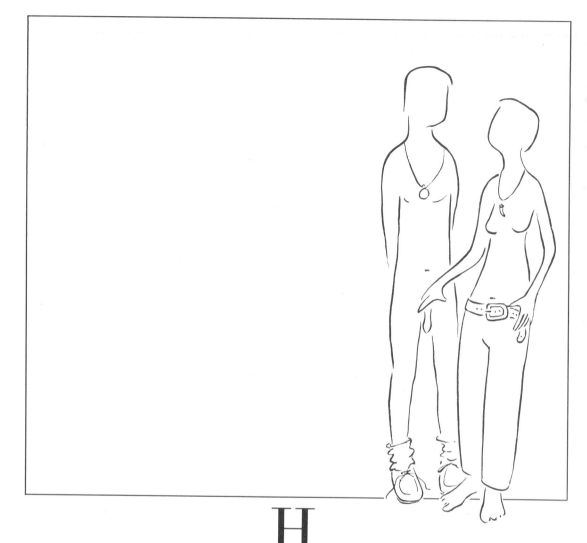

H e must
stand and obediently move as she may direct
so that she can enjoy looking at and touching his every part.
She may dress or undress him,
decorate him with jewelry, paint him with lipstick,
make him do calisthenics
or do anything that will intrigue and amuse her.
He may not touch her unless she gives him instructions,
but she can tantalize him without inhibitions.
If she chooses, she may use any part of him
such as a knee, a thumb or a big toe
to masturbate.

29

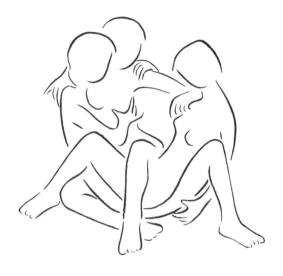

Т he Players
must devise their own Play.
It may be something they would like to do
that was not included in this book;
it may be anything
special
that is required by their fantasy or roles,
or
it may be a necessary adjustment
to accommodate other Players
who have been invited
to join in the Game.

30

PLAYERS
PICK
ONE
POSITION
AND
CONSUMMATE
THE
GAME
IN
THAT
POSITION

POSITIONS

FOR
USE
WHEN
PLAYING
EITHER
ROLE
OR
SITUATION
FANTASEX

PLAYERS
PICK
ONE
POSITION
AND
CONSUMMATE
THE
GAME
IN
THAT
POSITION

POSITIONS

FOR
USE
WHEN
PLAYING
EITHER
ROLE
OR
SITUATION
FANTASEX

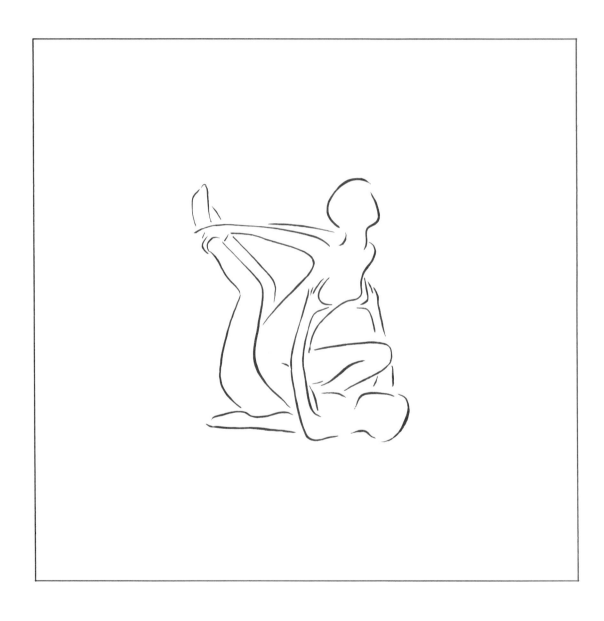

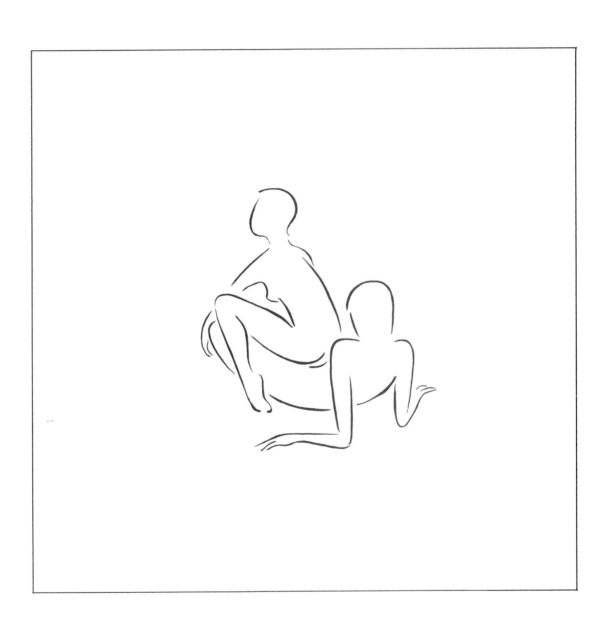

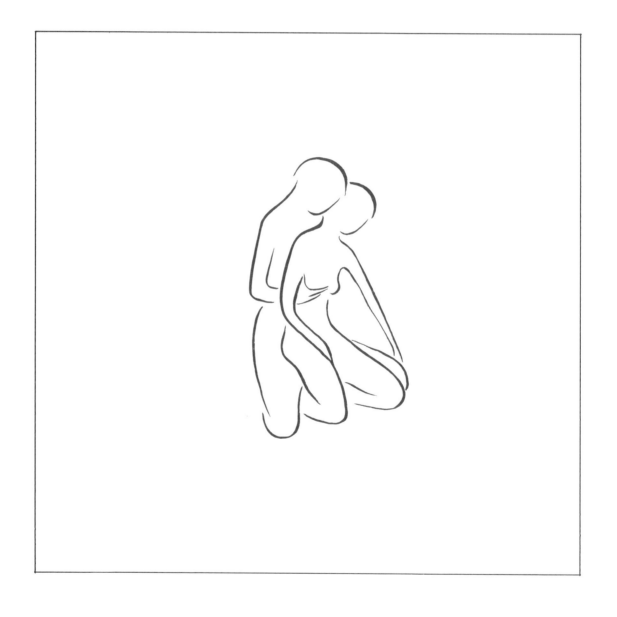

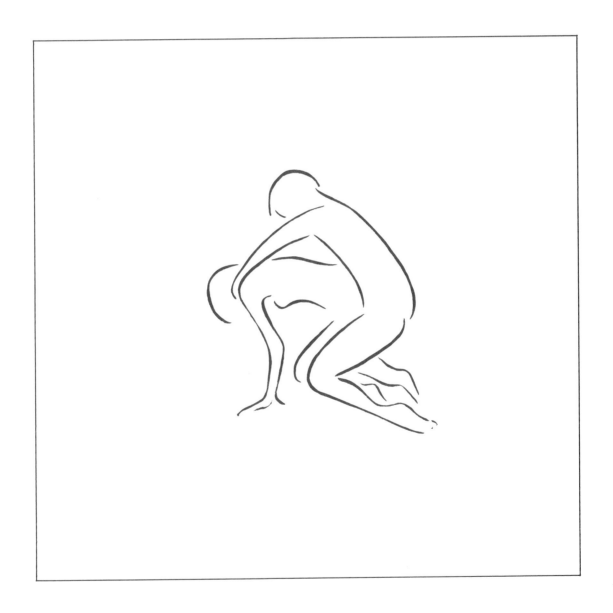

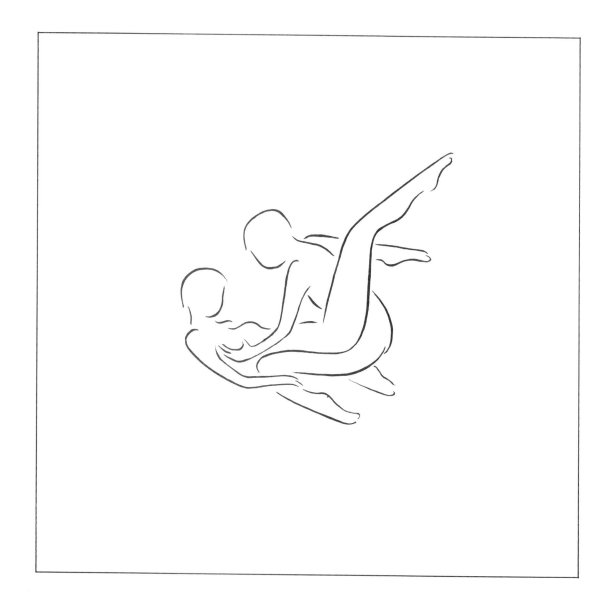

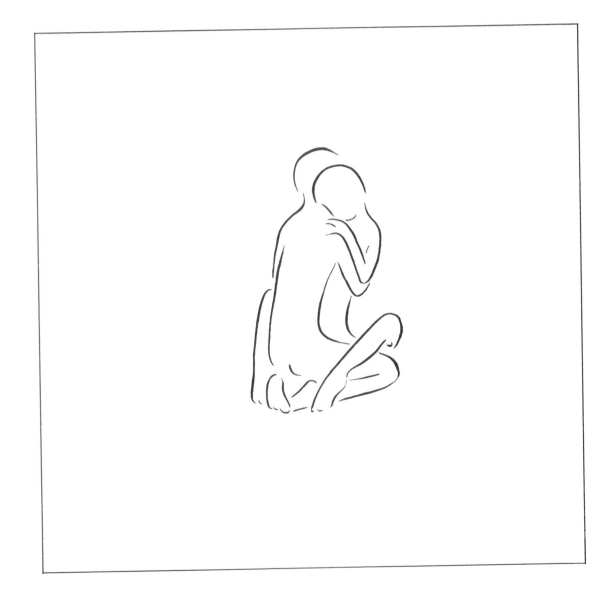

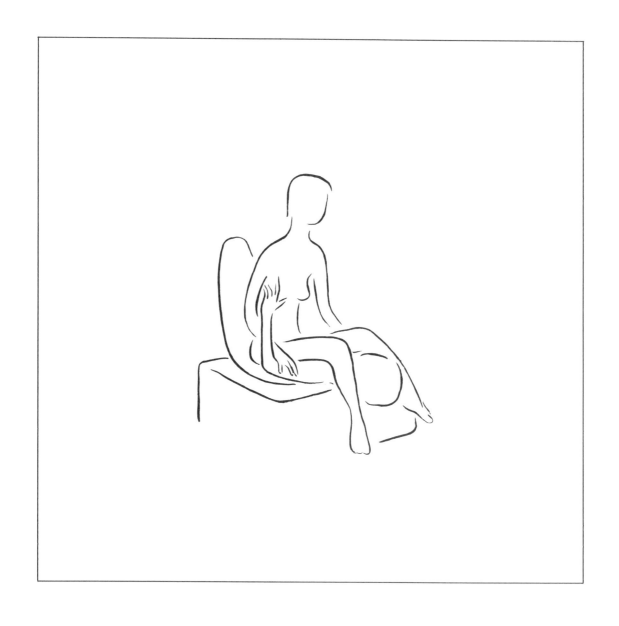

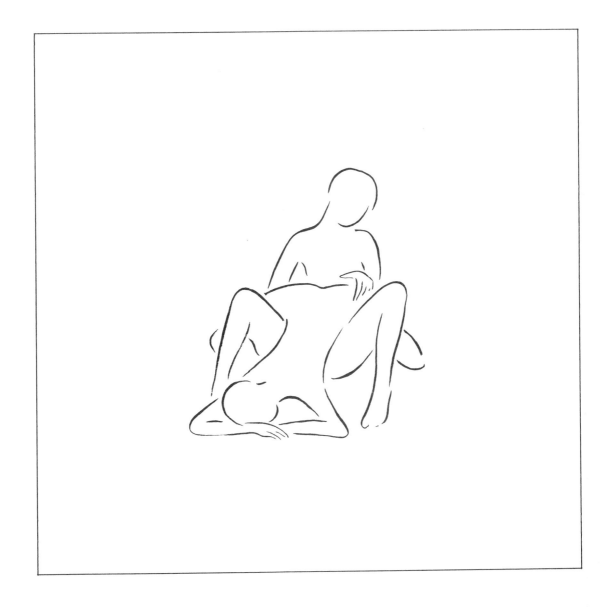

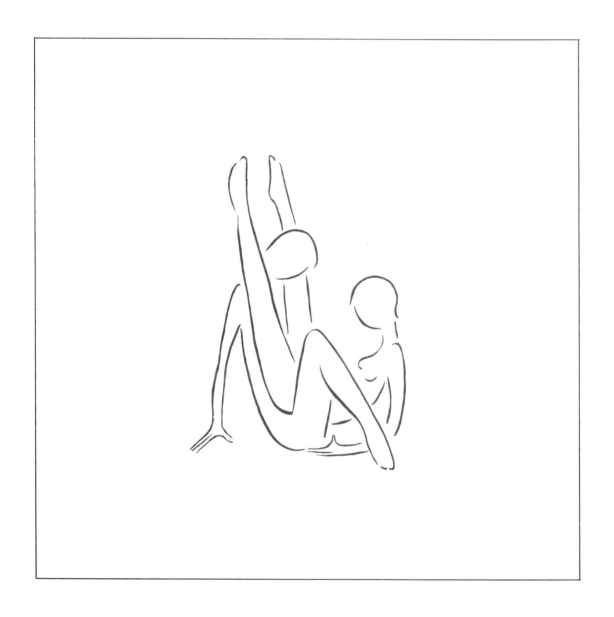

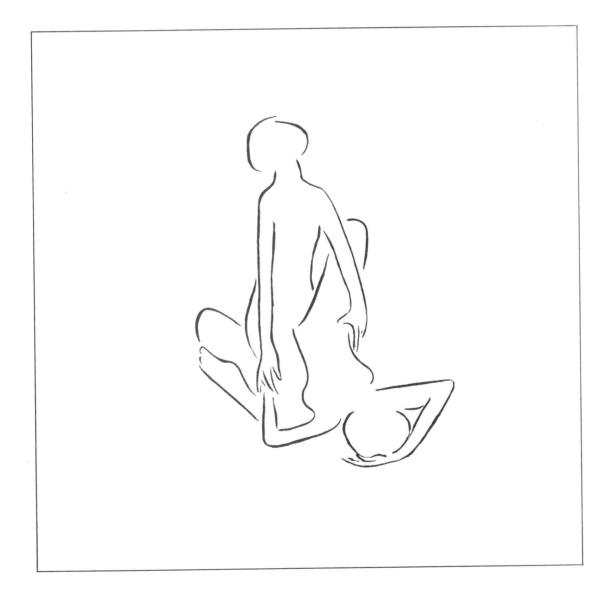

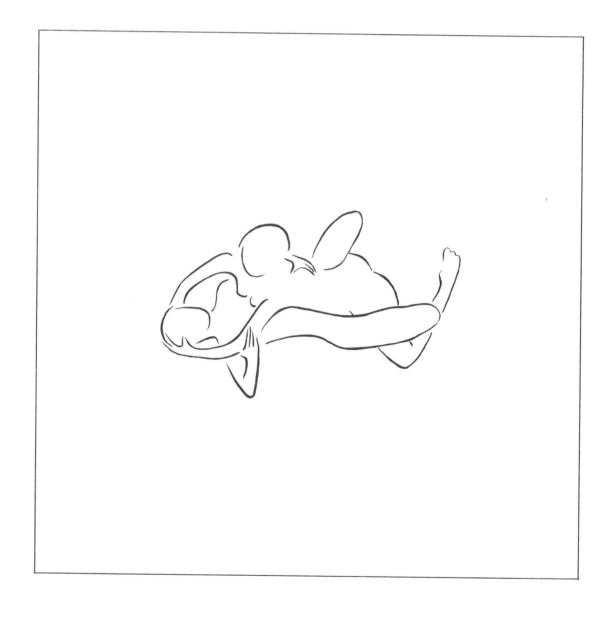

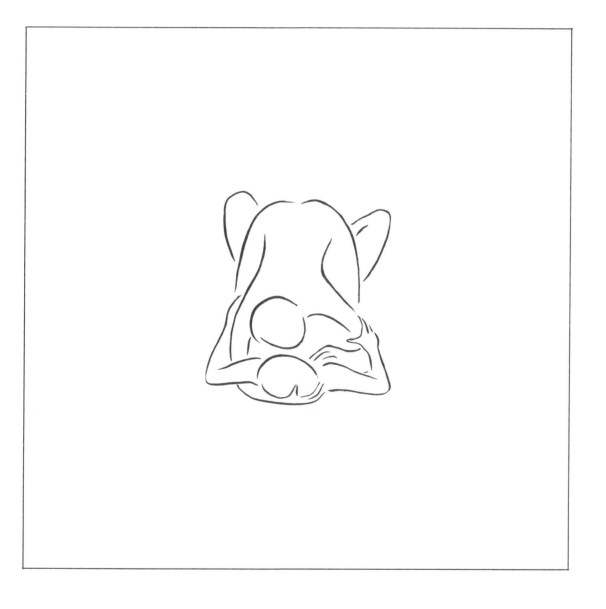

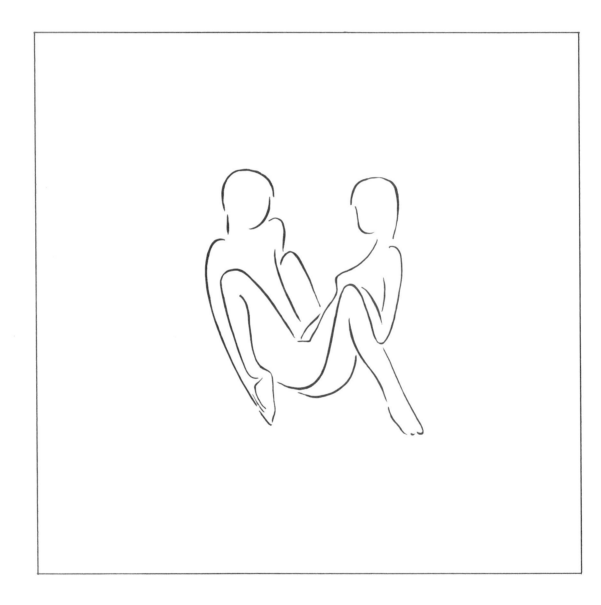

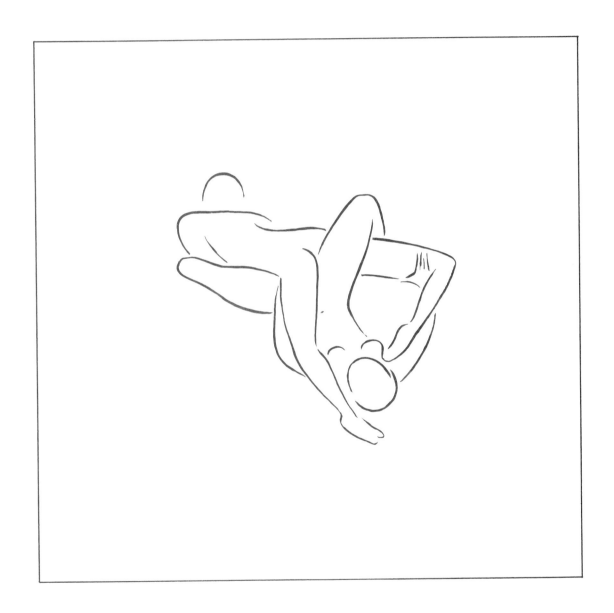

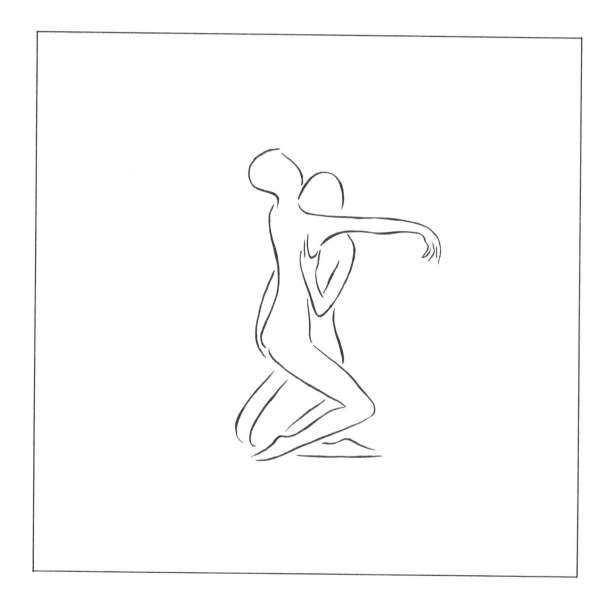

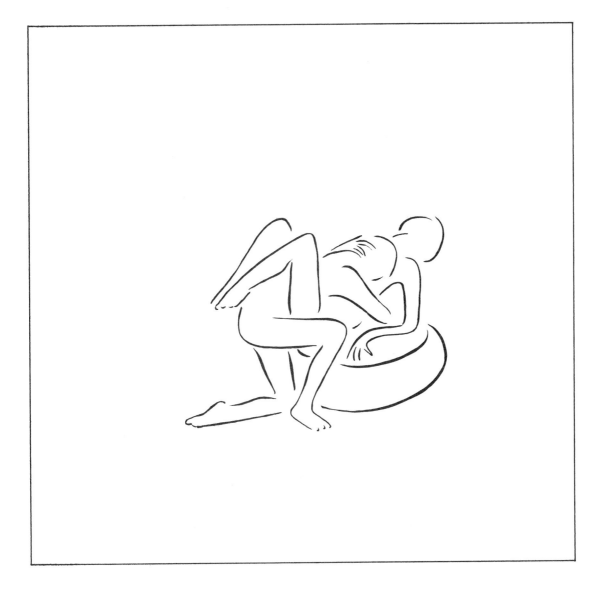

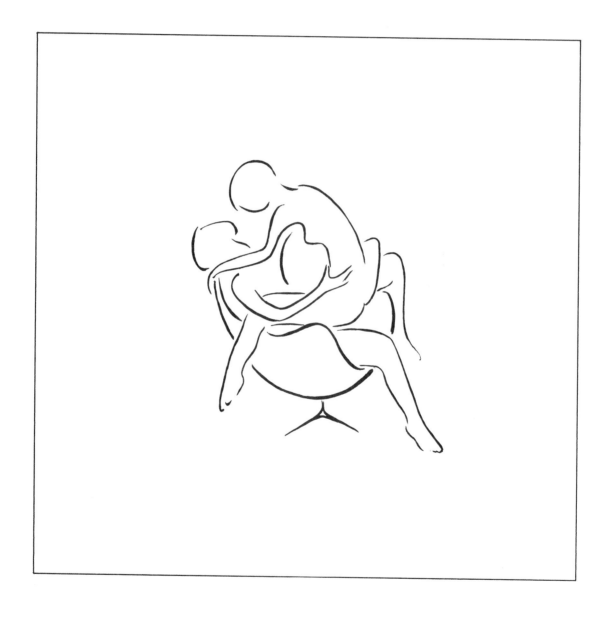

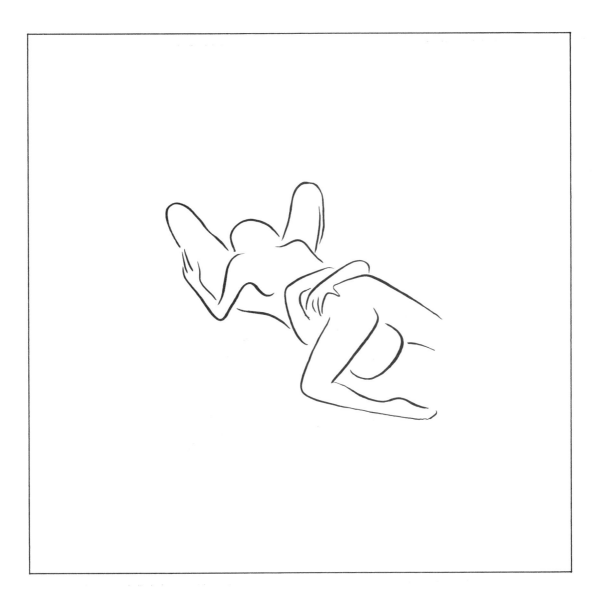

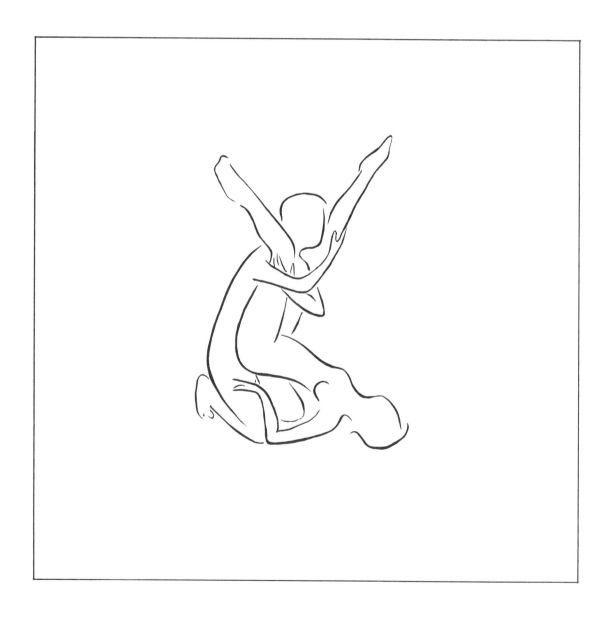

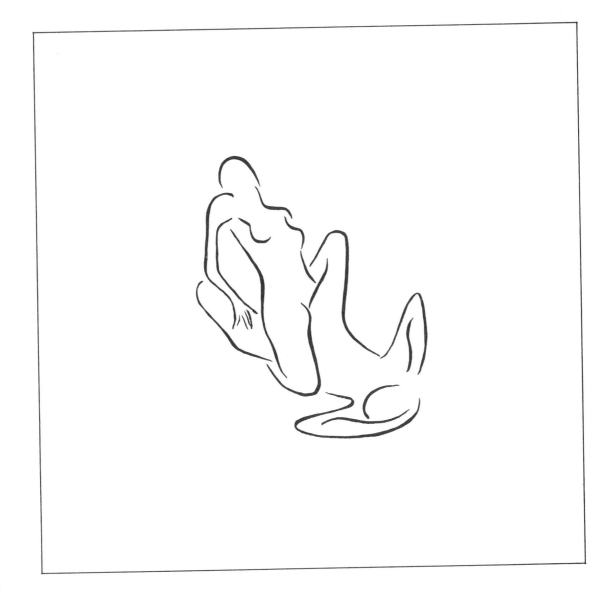

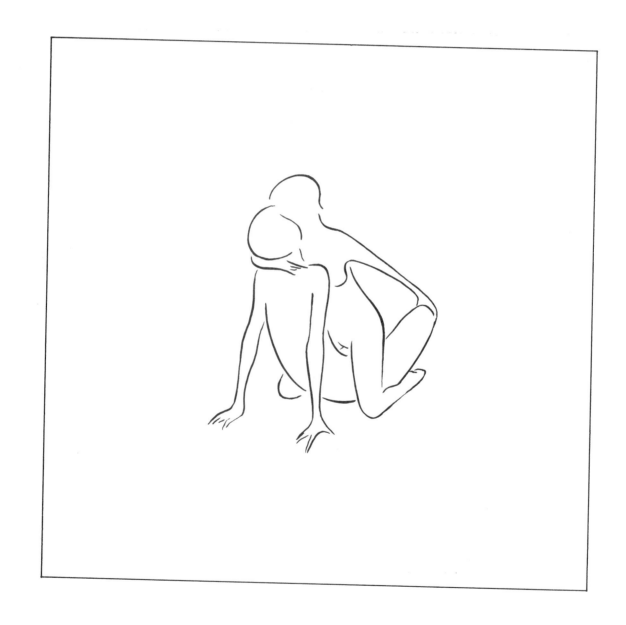

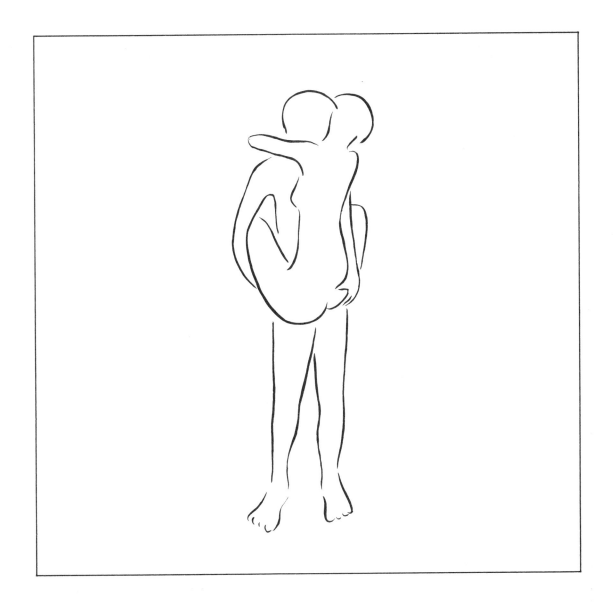

INSTRUCTIONS FOR PLAYING SITUATION FANTASEX

THE SECTIONS OF THE BOOK

As you know, the book is divided into several sections which can be easily recognized by leafing through. For the game of Situation Fantasex, the Players use the sections entitled "Fantasies," "Plays" and "Positions."

THE FANTASIES

A number of fantasy situations are described in the "Fantasies" section of the book. Since only one Fantasy can be developed and played during any one game, the Players read through the group and select the one they wish to use for the game.

They make the selection together in the Cooperative Game Plan. If they have chosen a Male or Female Dominant Game Plan, one Player will decide without consulting the other. If the Players have chosen the Pure Chance Game Plan, either Player picks a number from 1 to 40; they must then find the corresponding number in the "Fantasies" section of the book, and proceed with that Fantasy.

The specific situation will set the theme of the make-believe setting and relationship into which the Players will project themselves during the rest of the game.

FANTASIES

THE PLAYS

With the fantasy established, the Players should consult the "Plays" section of the book. From these, Players following the Cooperative Game Plan each select at least *one* Play. If they have chosen a Male or Female Dominant Game Plan, one Player will choose at least *two* Plays. If the Players have chosen the Pure Chance Game Plan, each Player picks a number from 1 to 30. They must then find the corresponding numbers in the "Plays" section of the book, and proceed with those Plays.

During the course of the game, they will have to incorporate into their fantasy all the directions given, before they are permitted to end the game.

THE POSITIONS

Next, if they are playing the Cooperative Game Plan, either Player may choose any one Position from the Positions section of the book.

If they are playing the Male or Female Dominant Game Plan, one Player picks the Position.

If the Players have chosen the Pure Chance Game Plan, either Player may pick a number from 1 to 22. They must then find the corresponding number in the "Positions" section of the book, and proceed with that Position.

No matter which Game Plan has been played, the Position chosen is the one that must be followed to consummate the game.

THE PROCEDURE

If they wish, the Players may dress up or dress down, depending on their fantasy situation. In any case, when all the decisions have been made, the Players relax and perhaps have another glass of wine as they project themselves into their imaginary relationship. Fantasizing together, they expand on the given theme as they make the transition from the real world to the world of make-believe and begin playing the game.

FOR
USE
WHEN
PLAYING
THE
SITUATION
FANTASEX
GAME

FANTASIES

PLAYERS
SELECT
AND
USE
ONE
SITUATION
ONLY

FANTASY

1

He caught her
skipping
through a lonely wooded glen.

They play together
whimsically

FANTASY

2

Unbeknownst to him
she has switched places with a 16-year-old virgin
for whom he has paid dearly.

She plays with him
deceptively

FANTASY

3

They met
in a strange hotel while traveling alone;
after tonight, they will never see each other again.

They play together
without inhibition

FANTASY

4

Their old-fashioned father keeps her from dating,
but doesn't suspect her brother
who is consoling her in her room.

He plays with her
fraternally

5

She will make him respond to her
even though he has never
made it with a woman before.

She plays with him
encouragingly

6

Her honor is being saved
for the wedding to her intended,
but she secretly meets the man she really loves.

They play together
romantically

7

They are aware that many others
are patiently standing in line,
waiting their turn.

They play together
lazily

8

She has just acquired him
at a slave auction
and is now evaluating her purchase.

He plays with her
obediently

9

Unbeknownst to her
he has switched places
with his identical twin brother.

He plays with her
schemingly

10

He surprised her
as she was currying the black stallion;
the snorting beast watches.

She plays with him
vicariously

11

They have instructions to practice
before they are sent into space together
to do it in the interest of science.

They play with each other
weightlessly

12

The authorities have selected her
for impregnation, and she has been given
to the racially pure hero for this purpose.

He plays with her
purposefully

FANTASY

13

He will make her respond to him
even though she has never
made it with a man.

He plays with her
patiently

FANTASY

14

The audience will demand their money back
unless pleased and excited
by their performance on the lighted stage.

They play together
dramatically

On her honeymoon cruise
while her husband is playing monopoly,
a dark stranger invites her to his cabin.

She plays with him
nervously

Programmed by a mad and greedy scientist
to give pleasure to whoever will rent their bodies,
they are waiting for a new assignment.

They play with each other
mechanically

17

He has saved her from drowning
and has brought her
to his cottage, which overlooks the lonely beach.

She plays with him
gratefully

18

It's another three years in solitary
unless he submits to the Warden's attentions;
she takes the Warden's role.

They play together
pretendingly

She is risking her life
to spend this moment with him;
for him, however, she is a one-night stand.

He plays with her
selfishly

They have been matched
by a quack sex therapist
to overcome their shyness and their shame.

They play together
impersonally

21

Each is married to another
but they have admired each other for ages from afar;
finally they are alone.

They play together
expressively

22

On the way to be wed to a repulsive prince,
her ship is captured by a handsome pirate
who deflowers the noble girl.

She plays with
mixed emotions

He is inexperienced
and she has undertaken the project
to teach him about love.

She plays with him
instructively

With his Oriental inscrutability
her host spiked the drinks
with an effective aphrodisiac.

They play together
uncontrollably

25

He is her social inferior
and even though her family is mortified,
she feels a moral obligation.

They play together
democratically

26

She has taken him to the attic
where the soundproofed walls are decorated
with whips and chains and harnesses.

She plays with him
aggressively

FANTASY

27

Following the doctor's posthypnotic suggestion,
the beast in her is freed,
and she forgets all she believed was proper.

Liberated at last
she enjoys the ridiculous games

FANTASY

28

She has been unable to give him an heir;
his people demand
that he leave her and marry another.

They play together
tragically

FANTASY
29

This is their last night together
for they both know
that she has only a few days to live.

They play together
tenderly

FANTASY
30

They need a sorority mascot;
she checks his qualifications
as her sisters watch them through a one-way mirror.

She plays with him
experimentally

31

Her lover has taken her to his men's club
where he induces her to submit to a friend
while he enjoys watching.

They play together
lasciviously

32

His career will be ruined
by this tryst;
however, he feels that he cannot resist her.

He plays with her
insatiably

FANTASY
33

He is a host at a health spa
where he has to massage his rich client;
his tip depends on how well he pleases her.

He plays with her
professionally

FANTASY
34

Unaware that she has idolized him for years,
he invites her for drinks
in his fabulous penthouse apartment.

He plays with her
matter-of-factly

35

She will be fired from the job she needs
if she will not submit to her lesbian employer;
he takes the boss's role.

They play together
pretendingly

36

She has betrayed him
and knows that they will kill him
as he leaves the house.

She plays with him in
anticipation

37

They abandon their respective lovers
at the crowded church reception, and
go to the privacy of the quiet chapel.

They play together
adulterously

38

She is directing an X-rated movie.
Working with her star performer,
she explores new angles.

They play together
dirtily

39

While studying the habits
of a remote jungle tribe, she finds herself
all alone with the ruling prince.

They play together
curiously

40

She is the vestal virgin
whom the Priest has chosen to initiate
on the altar in the candlelit cave.

He plays with her
ceremoniously

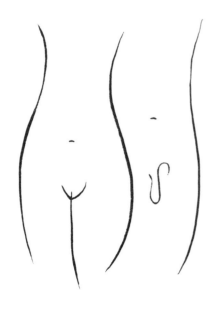